UNRAVELING THE SPECTRUM

Embracing The Brilliance Of Autism

BY

LAURA WARREN, M.D

Table of Contents

Introduction

Chapter 1
Understanding Autism Spectrum Disorder

Chapter 2
Early Signs and Diagnosis: Identifying Autism

Chapter 3
Inside the Autistic Mind: Perception and Sensory Processing

Chapter 4
Communication Challenges and Breakthroughs

Chapter 5
Navigating Social Interactions: Building Connections

Chapter 6
Unveiling Hidden Talents: Embracing Strengths in Autism

Chapter 7
Therapies and Interventions: Enhancing Quality of Life

Chapter 8
Family Support and Advocacy: The Journey Together

Chapter 9
Education and Inclusion: Creating Supportive Environments

Chapter 10
Empowering Autistic Individuals: Embracing Diversity in Society

Conclusion

Introduction

Autism, also known as Autism Spectrum Disorder (ASD), is a complex neurodevelopmental condition that affects communication, behavior, and social interaction. It is characterized by a wide range of challenges and strengths, leading to a spectrum of symptoms that vary in severity from person to person.

Individuals with autism may experience difficulties in understanding social cues, expressing emotions, and forming meaningful relationships. However, they often demonstrate unique talents and abilities in areas like art, mathematics, music, or memorization.

Early diagnosis and intervention play a crucial role in helping individuals with autism lead fulfilling lives. While there is currently no cure for autism, various therapies and support systems can help improve communication skills, behavior, and overall quality of life for those affected.

It is important to promote awareness and understanding of autism to create a more inclusive and accepting society. By embracing diversity and recognizing the strengths of individuals on the autism spectrum, we can foster a world that values the unique contributions of every individual.

Chapter 1

Understanding Autism Spectrum Disorder

Autism Spectrum Disorder (ASD) is a neurodevelopmental disorder that affects communication, behavior, and social interaction. It is characterized by a wide range of symptoms and severity levels, which is why it's called a "spectrum." Individuals with ASD may have challenges with verbal and nonverbal communication, repetitive behaviors, and difficulties in understanding social cues.

The exact cause of ASD is not fully understood, but both genetic and environmental factors are believed to play a role. Early diagnosis and intervention can significantly improve the quality of life for individuals with ASD, helping them develop coping skills and reach their full potential. It's important to approach each person with understanding, support, and acceptance, recognizing their unique strengths and challenges.

Here are some more details about Autism Spectrum Disorder (ASD):

Symptoms and Characteristics

ASD can manifest in a variety of ways, and its symptoms typically appear in early childhood. Common signs include challenges in social interaction and communication, restricted interests, repetitive behaviors, and sensory sensitivities. Some individuals may have difficulty maintaining eye contact, using gestures, or understanding non- literal language such as sarcasm.

Diagnosis

ASD is typically diagnosed in childhood, often around the age of 2 to 3 years, though some cases may be diagnosed earlier or later. Diagnosing ASD involves a comprehensive evaluation by healthcare professionals, including pediatricians, psychologists, and developmental specialists. Observations of behavior, interviews with parents/caregivers, and standardized assessments are used to assess communication skills, social behavior, and repetitive behaviors.

Autism Spectrum

ASD is often referred to as a "spectrum" because the severity and impact of symptoms can vary widely among individuals. Some people may have mild challenges and be highly functional, while others may require more support in daily living.

Causes of ASD

The exact causes of ASD remain unknown, but research suggests a combination of genetic and environmental factors. Certain genetic mutations and prenatal factors may increase the risk of developing ASD, but it's important to note that not all cases can be linked to specific causes.

Interventions and Support

Early intervention is crucial for children with ASD to promote development and adaptive skills. Applied Behavior Analysis (ABA) therapy, speech therapy, occupational therapy, and social skills training are commonly used to address specific challenges.

As a behaviorist, we look at behavior functions before determining the reasons why behavior excess or deficit continue to happen. After a functional assessment, some of the following may be implemented.

For adolescent and up- Program to Teach;
- Shaping
- Chaining
- Prompts
- Extinction
- Set and follow routines
- Reinforcement
- Reduce Novelty
- Eliminate triggers

For toddlers and up- Program to Develop;

- Problem solving
- Sorting, matching
- Recall
- Bin in room
- Checklist
- Goal setting
- Visual schedule
- Provide Template

Co-occurring Conditions

Many individuals with ASD may also have other co-occurring conditions, such as intellectual disabilities, attention deficit hyperactivity disorder (ADHD), anxiety, or epilepsy.

Treatment and Management

There is no cure for ASD, but various interventions and therapies can significantly improve an individual's quality of life. Applied Behavior Analysis (ABA), speech therapy, occupational therapy, and social skills training are commonly used approaches.

Support for Families

Families of individuals with ASD may face unique challenges. Support groups and counseling can be beneficial in helping parents and caregivers navigate the complexities of raising a child with ASD.

Transition to Adulthood

As individuals with ASD grow into adulthood, they may need support in transitioning to independent living, vocational training, and employment opportunities suited to their strengths and interests.

Awareness and Acceptance

Raising awareness and promoting acceptance of individuals with ASD are essential to creating an inclusive and supportive society. Remember that each person with ASD is unique, and understanding and empathy are essential in providing appropriate support and care. It's also essential to consult with

healthcare professionals or specialists for
personalized information and guidance.

Chapter 2

Early Signs and Diagnosis: Identifying Autism

Early signs of autism can vary, but they may include
limited eye contact, delayed speech and language
skills, repetitive behaviors, difficulty with social
interactions, and intense interests in specific topics.

Diagnosis typically involves observing a child's
behavior and development, along with assessments
conducted by healthcare professionals and

specialists in autism. Early identification and intervention are crucial for better outcomes because early intervention can significantly improve the child's development and overall quality of life. If you have concerns, consult a pediatrician or a developmental specialist.

Here are some early signs of autism that parents, caregivers, and healthcare professionals may look for in infants and toddlers:

1. Social Communication Difficulties: A child might avoid eye contact, not respond to their name being called, or have trouble understanding nonverbal cues like facial expressions.

2. Language and Communication Challenges: Delayed or absent speech and language skills are common in children with autism. They may also repeat words or phrases (echolalia) without understanding their meaning.

3. Repetitive Behaviors: Children with autism may engage in repetitive movements, like rocking or

hand-flapping. They might also have intense interests in specific topics, objects, or activities.

4. Social Interaction Difficulties: Difficulty in forming relationships with peers, trouble sharing interests or emotions, and challenges in understanding social rules and norms.

5. Sensory Sensitivities: Some children with autism may have heightened or reduced sensitivity to sensory inputs like light, sound, textures, or smells.

6. Red Flags for Autism: Early identification of autism can be challenging, as some behaviors might be present in typically developing children as well. However, certain "red flags" can signal the need for further evaluation. These red flags include:

- Lack of pointing or gesturing by 12 months.
- No babbling or using single words by 16 months.
- No two-word phrases by 24 months.
- Loss of previously acquired language.

7. Limited Interests: Children with autism may show intense focus on specific topics or objects, often to the exclusion of other activities or toys. They may display repetitive play patterns that center around these interests.

8. Diagnostic Process: The diagnostic process for autism typically involves a multidisciplinary team of professionals, which may include pediatricians, child psychologists, developmental specialists, speech and language therapists, and occupational therapists. The process generally includes the following steps:

9. Developmental Screening: This is often the first step in identifying autism. Pediatricians may use standardized screening tools to assess a child's development and identify any potential red flags.

10. Comprehensive Evaluation: A thorough evaluation involves observing the child's behavior and interactions, gathering information from parents and caregivers about the child's developmental history, and conducting various assessments to

evaluate speech, language, cognitive, social, and motor skills.

11. Diagnostic Criteria: The diagnosis of autism is based on criteria outlined in the DSM-5 (Diagnostic and Statistical Manual of Mental Disorders, 5th Edition) or the ICD-10/ICD-11 (International Classification of Diseases).

12. Medical Evaluation: A medical evaluation is essential to rule out other medical conditions that may present similar symptoms to autism.

13. Early Intervention: Early intervention is critical for children with autism, as it can significantly improve their developmental outcomes and long-term functioning. Interventions are tailored to the individual needs of each child and may include:

14. Behavioral Therapies:Applied Behavior Analysis (ABA) is a commonly used therapy that focuses on reinforcing positive behaviors and reducing problematic ones. It helps children develop communication, social, and daily living skills.

15. Speech and Language Therapy: This therapy addresses communication challenges and helps children improve their verbal and nonverbal communication skills.

16. Occupational Therapy: Occupational therapy helps children develop fine motor skills, self-care abilities, and sensory processing.

17. Educational Support: Special education programs can provide a structured learning environment tailored to a child's specific needs.

18. Parent Training and Support: Parents play a crucial role in their child's development, so training and support services are essential to help them understand and manage their child's needs effectively.

Chapter 3

Inside the Autistic Mind: Perception and Sensory Processing

Understanding the autistic mind's perception and sensory processing can shed light on the unique sensory experiences individuals with autism may have. Sensory processing refers to how the brain receives and interprets sensory information from the environment. In autism, sensory processing differences can be significant and affect various senses, such as sight, sound, touch, taste, and smell.

It's important to note that sensory experiences can vary widely among autistic individuals. Each person may have their unique sensory profile, and what might be overwhelming for one individual may be soothing or neutral for another.

Understanding sensory processing in autism can help create more accommodating and supportive environments. By recognizing and respecting these differences, caregivers, educators, and society as a whole can better support individuals with autism and enhance their quality of life. Occupational therapy and sensory integration techniques can be beneficial in addressing sensory challenges and promoting self-regulation.

1. Sensory Overload and Meltdowns:
Sensory overload occurs when the brain receives more sensory information than it can process effectively. In autistic individuals, this can lead to meltdowns, which are intense reactions to overwhelming stimuli.

Meltdowns are not tantrums; they are involuntary responses to distress. During a meltdown, individuals may become highly agitated, irritable, or even exhibit self-injurious behaviors. Providing a quiet and safe space during meltdowns can be essential for the person to calm down and regulate their sensory experiences.

2. Sensory Under-Responsiveness and Safety Concerns: Sensory under-responsiveness can lead to

safety concerns, as individuals may not react appropriately to potentially dangerous situations. For example, they might not respond to pain or temperature changes, which can increase the risk of accidents or injuries. Caregivers need to be attentive to these issues and ensure the individual's safety in various environments.

3. Repetitive Behaviors as Sensory Regulation: Repetitive behaviors, known as stimming, are common in autism and can serve as a way to self-regulate sensory experiences. Examples of stimming include hand-flapping, rocking, finger-flicking, or repetitive vocalizations. These behaviors help individuals cope with sensory overload or provide comfort in stressful situations.

4. Auditory Processing Challenges: Many autistic individuals have auditory processing challenges, making it challenging to filter or prioritize sounds. Noises that might be background noise to neurotypical individuals can be overwhelming and distracting for those with autism. This can impact their ability to focus, follow

instructions, or participate in conversations, especially in noisy environments.

5. Visual Processing Differences and Hyperfocus: Some autistic individuals experience hyperfocus, where they become deeply engrossed in specific tasks or subjects. This intense focus can be an asset in certain areas but may also lead to difficulties shifting attention to other tasks or social interactions.

6. Sensory Sensitivities and Challenges in Daily Life: Sensory sensitivities can impact various aspects of daily life. For example, individuals may struggle with clothing choices due to fabric textures, have aversions to specific food textures, or avoid certain environments because of overwhelming sensory stimuli. Understanding these sensitivities and making appropriate accommodations can help reduce anxiety and improve the individual's well-being.

7. Sensory-Friendly Environments:
Creating sensory-friendly environments is crucial
for supporting autistic individuals. Reducing harsh
lighting, minimizing noise, providing sensory toys,
and offering quiet spaces for breaks can make a
significant difference. Sensory-friendly strategies in
schools, workplaces, and public spaces can promote
inclusivity and reduce sensory overload.

8. Sensory Preferences and Avoidance:
Autistic individuals may have specific sensory
preferences, where they seek out or enjoy particular
sensations. For example, some may enjoy deep
pressure, seeking hugs or heavy blankets for
comfort. On the other hand, they might actively
avoid sensory experiences they find distressing, such
as covering their ears to block out loud noises.

9. Unpredictable Sensory Reactions:
Sensory reactions in autism can be unpredictable
and may vary based on factors like fatigue, stress, or
the individual's emotional state. Something that was
tolerable on one occasion might trigger sensory
overload on another day. This variability can

sometimes lead to challenges in predicting and managing sensory responses.

10. Sensory Processing Disorder (SPD) and Co-Occurring Conditions: Sensory Processing Disorder (SPD) is not an officially diagnosed disorder, but doctors and other professionals who work with autistic patients often use the term. Sensory processing challenges in autism can sometimes be part of a broader condition called Sensory Processing Disorder (SPD).

 SPD is not a standalone diagnosis in the DSM-5 (Diagnostic and Statistical Manual of Mental Disorders, Version-5) criteria, which states that **hyper - or hypo reactivity(an exaggerated or minimized response) to environment stimuli** , or an unusual interest in them may be a sign of autism, but it is recognized by some practitioners and researchers. Some individuals with autism may have co-occurring SPD, which can intensify sensory experiences and responses.

11. Coping Mechanisms and Self-Regulation: Autistic individuals develop various coping mechanisms to manage sensory input and regulate their responses. These coping strategies can be constructive or potentially harmful, depending on their nature. Encouraging positive and safe self-regulation techniques, such as deep breathing exercises or using sensory toys, can be beneficial.

12. Sensory Integration Therapy: Sensory Integration Therapy is a specialized intervention designed to help individuals with sensory processing difficulties. The therapy aims to improve the brain's ability to process and integrate sensory information effectively. It involves engaging the individual in activities that challenge their sensory systems in a structured and supportive environment.

13. Multisensory Approaches to Learning: For autistic individuals, incorporating multisensory approaches to learning can enhance their educational experiences. Utilizing visual aids, hands-on activities, and auditory cues can facilitate better understanding and retention of information.

14. Sensory Sensitivities and Anxiety:
Sensory sensitivities can contribute to heightened anxiety levels in autistic individuals. Being in sensory-rich environments or facing sensory triggers may lead to increased stress and difficulties in managing emotions. Recognizing these triggers and implementing anxiety-reduction strategies can be valuable in promoting emotional well-being.

15. Empowering Autistic Individuals:
Empowering autistic individuals to communicate their sensory needs and preferences is crucial. Encouraging open dialogue and active listening can help caregivers and educators understand how sensory experiences impact each individual uniquely.

16. Sensory Profiles and Individualized Support:
Every autistic person has a distinct sensory profile. Some may have heightened sensitivity in one sensory area while being under-responsive in another. Recognizing these profiles and providing individualized support is essential to address specific challenges effectively.

On the other hand, autistic individuals may also exhibit sensory avoidance. They might be highly sensitive to certain stimuli and actively try to avoid them. This could include avoiding crowded or noisy places, wearing specific clothing materials, or reacting adversely to strong smells. Avoidance behaviors can help them manage sensory overload and maintain a sense of control in their environment.

Executive Function Deficits

1. Organizational

2. Attention problem

3. Inhibition

4. Classroom/ home issues

5. Problem solving

Organizational

- Arriving late
- Not completing task
- Not enough time
- No plans for what to do
- Losing things

Attention Problem

- Trouble focusing
- Distracted
- Does not complete task

Inhibition

- Acts on impulse
- Unaware of things that annoy others
- Does not stop when told to stop
- Talking too loud
- Nail biting

Classroom/Home Issues

- Untidy room
- Littered toys
- Aggression
- Not attending classes
- Task disruption
- Distraction

Problem Solving

- Forgetting things
- Always asking for help
- Tries same solution for all problems
- Not learning from mistakes
- Difficulty completing simple tasks

Collaborating with occupational therapists and other sensory specialists can be valuable in identifying sensory profiles and developing individualized strategies to address sensory challenges. The goal is to create environments and experiences that support and enhance each person's strengths while accommodating their sensory differences.

However, perception and sensory processing are essential aspects of the autistic mind. Understanding and embracing these differences can lead to more inclusive and supportive environments that empower autistic individuals to thrive and participate fully in society. By recognizing the individuality of sensory experiences and providing targeted interventions, we can promote a more inclusive and enriching world for everyone.

Understanding perception and sensory processing in autism goes beyond simply acknowledging differences. It involves recognizing that sensory experiences play a significant role in the lives of autistic individuals and can profoundly impact their well-being, behavior, and social interactions. By promoting sensory-friendly environments, offering targeted interventions, and respecting individual preferences, we can create more inclusive and supportive communities for people with autism.

Perception and sensory processing play a vital role in the experiences of autistic individuals. Understanding and accommodating sensory differences can lead to improved well-being, increased participation in daily activities, and better social interactions. By embracing neurodiversity and recognizing the uniqueness of each individual's sensory profile, we can foster a more inclusive and supportive society for everyone.

Chapter 4

Communication Challenges and Breakthroughs

Communication is an essential aspect of human interaction, enabling the exchange of ideas, emotions, and information. However, various challenges can hinder effective communication, leading to misunderstandings and conflicts.

Some common communication challenges include language barriers, cultural differences, and misinterpretations. Language barriers can impede understanding when individuals speak different languages or struggle with technical jargon. Cultural differences, such as norms and nonverbal cues, can also lead to misunderstandings.

Moreover, technological advancements have introduced new challenges, like communication overload and miscommunication in digital platforms. The prevalence of distractions and multitasking can disrupt meaningful conversations, making it difficult to convey messages accurately.

However, amidst these challenges, breakthroughs have emerged to enhance communication. Advancements in translation technology have bridged language gaps, making it easier for people from diverse backgrounds to communicate. Furthermore, improved audio and video conferencing tools have fostered remote communication, connecting people across the globe seamlessly.

In addition, social media and instant messaging platforms have provided convenient channels for exchanging information quickly. Though these platforms pose challenges in terms of privacy and misinformation, they have also enabled individuals to connect and share ideas in real-time.

Overall, as communication challenges persist, continuous breakthroughs in technology and cross-cultural understanding have the potential to revolutionize the way we interact, bringing people closer and promoting effective communication in an increasingly interconnected world.

However, there are few communication challenges below;

1. Language barriers: Overcoming differences in languages can be a significant obstacle to effective communication.

2. Misinterpretation: Messages can be misunderstood or misinterpreted, leading to confusion and conflicts.

3. Lack of active listening: Failure to listen actively can result in missed information and poor understanding.

4. Cultural differences: Different cultural norms and communication styles may lead to misunderstandings and offense.

5. Non-verbal cues: Interpreting body language and facial expressions can be challenging, especially in virtual communication.

Communication Breakthroughs;

1. Advancements in technology: Tools like instant messaging, video conferencing, and AI translation have improved global communication.

2. Cross-cultural training: Organizations and individuals are investing in training to understand and appreciate diverse cultures.

3. Emotional intelligence: Greater emphasis on emotional intelligence helps people understand and empathize with others' perspectives.

4. Visual aids and multimedia: Using images, videos, and graphics enhances communication and makes complex ideas easier to grasp.

5. Collaboration platforms: Online platforms that allow real-time collaboration enable seamless communication between teams and individuals. In face-to-face interactions, these cues add depth and context to the message.

However, in virtual communication or written correspondence, these cues may be absent, leading to potential misunderstandings. Emoticons or emoji can partially compensate for this in digital communication, but it's essential to remain aware of the limitations and potential misinterpretations.

In essence, communication challenges are ever-present in our diverse and fast-paced world. However, breakthroughs in technology, cultural awareness, emotional intelligence, visual aids, and collaboration platforms are continuously transforming how we communicate, enabling more effective and meaningful interactions in various aspects of life and work.

Chapter 5

Navigating Social Interactions: Building Connections

Navigating social interactions and building connections involves understanding and respecting others' perspectives, actively listening, and finding common interests to engage in meaningful conversations. It also includes maintaining positive body language, expressing empathy, and being genuine in your interactions to foster authentic relationships with others. Remember, building connections is a continuous process that requires practice and openness to new experiences.

Building connections in social interactions involves several key factors. Here are some strategies to help you navigate and improve your social interactions:

1. Active Listening: Pay attention to what others are saying, show genuine interest, and respond appropriately. This demonstrates that you value their thoughts and feelings.

2. Empathy and Understanding: Try to put yourself in the other person's shoes, and be sensitive to their emotions and perspectives.

3. Positive Body Language: Maintain eye contact, smile, and use open and welcoming gestures to create a friendly atmosphere.

4. Find Common Interests: Discover shared hobbies or topics of interest to bond over and deepen your connection.

5. Be Authentic: Be true to yourself and share your thoughts and feelings honestly, which can foster trust and deeper connections.

6. Be Supportive: Offer encouragement and help when needed, showing that you care about the well-being of others.

7. Avoid Judgment: Be non-judgmental and open-minded, allowing people to feel comfortable being themselves around you.

8. Initiate Conversations: Take the initiative to start conversations with others, even if it feels outside your comfort zone.

9. Remember Names and Details: Pay attention to people's names and important details about their lives, as this shows you value their presence.

10. Give Compliments: Offer genuine compliments to make others feel appreciated and valued.

11. Respecting Boundaries: Be aware of personal space and emotional boundaries. Avoid prying into sensitive topics and always ask for consent before discussing potentially private matters.

12. Positive Reinforcement: Provide positive feedback and encouragement to others. A supportive attitude fosters a sense of comfort and trust.

Remember, building connections takes time and effort, but the rewards of meaningful friendships and strong social bonds are worth it. Be patient, open-minded, and willing to invest in your relationships.

Chapter 6

Unveiling Hidden Talents: Embracing Strengths in Autism

Embracing hidden talents in autism is a beautiful way to support individuals and help them thrive. Many people with autism possess unique strengths, such as exceptional memory, attention to detail, creativity, and a deep focus on specific interests. By recognizing and nurturing these talents, we can create a more inclusive and understanding society. Encouraging individuals with autism to explore their strengths can lead to personal growth and meaningful contributions to various fields. Let's celebrate diversity and appreciate the incredible abilities within the autism community.

Embracing Strengths in Autism" is a chapter that focuses on recognizing and harnessing the unique strengths and abilities found in individuals with autism. It aims to shed light on the positive aspects of autism and encourages a more inclusive approach to supporting individuals on the autism spectrum.

The chapter could begin by providing an overview of autism and its characteristics, emphasizing that autism is a neurodevelopmental disorder and not a disability. It's essential to break the stigma and misconceptions surrounding autism and highlight the diverse range of talents and strengths that individuals with autism can possess.

The chapter may delve into some common hidden talents frequently observed in individuals with autism. These may include:

1. Unique Strengths in Autism: People with autism often possess unique cognitive abilities and strengths due to the atypical brain development associated with the condition. These strengths can vary widely among individuals but commonly include:

- Enhanced Perceptual Abilities: Some autistic individuals may have heightened senses, such as increased visual or auditory perception, which can be advantageous in certain fields like art, music, or design.

- Pattern Recognition: Many individuals with autism exhibit exceptional pattern recognition skills, which can be beneficial in fields such as mathematics, science, and engineering.

- Memory: As mentioned earlier, some individuals with autism have excellent memory abilities, particularly in areas of personal interest or specific subjects.

- Attention to Detail: Autistic individuals often pay great attention to details, making them well-suited for tasks that require precision and accuracy.

- Intense Focus and Concentration: Individuals with autism might demonstrate an extraordinary ability to focus intensely on their areas of interest, leading to significant accomplishments in those fields.

2. Creativity and Unique Perspectives: Autistic individuals often have a different way of perceiving

the world, leading to innovative and creative thinking.

3. Hyperfocus: Some individuals with autism experience periods of hyperfocus, enabling them to achieve remarkable results in tasks they are passionate about.

4. Artistic Expression: Many individuals with autism find artistic expression to be a powerful outlet for their thoughts and emotions. Art, music, writing, and other forms of creativity can serve as valuable means of communication and self-expression for individuals on the autism spectrum.

5. Neurodiversity Advocacy: The concept of neurodiversity advocates for embracing neurological differences, including autism, as a valuable part of human diversity. This perspective promotes acceptance, understanding, and support for individuals with autism, recognizing the strengths they bring to society.

The chapter could also emphasize the importance of creating an inclusive environment that encourages the exploration and development of these talents. This involves fostering acceptance, providing appropriate support, and accommodating individual needs.

Furthermore, it could discuss the significance of early intervention and support in identifying and nurturing these strengths from a young age. Encouragement from parents, teachers, and peers can play a crucial role in boosting confidence and self-esteem.

Additionally, the chapter may highlight real-life success stories of individuals with autism who have embraced their strengths and made significant contributions in various fields like arts, technology, mathematics, and more. These stories can serve as inspiring examples of how society can benefit from embracing diversity and celebrating the talents within the autism community.

In summary, embracing strengths in autism involves recognizing the diverse talents that individuals on the autism spectrum possess and providing supportive environments that nurture their abilities.

By celebrating neurodiversity and fostering
inclusive practices, we can create a society where
everyone has the opportunity to thrive and
contribute their unique gifts.

Chapter 7

Therapies and Interventions: Enhancing Quality of Life

Therapies and interventions can play a crucial role in enhancing the quality of life for individuals. These can vary depending on the specific needs and conditions of the person involved. Some common approaches include:

1. Physical Therapy: This therapy is beneficial for individuals with injuries, disabilities, or medical conditions affecting their movement and function. A physical therapist assesses the person's condition and develops a personalized treatment plan, including exercises, stretches, and manual techniques, to improve strength, flexibility, balance, and coordination. Physical therapy can help people regain independence and reduce pain.

2. Occupational Therapy: Occupational therapists focus on helping individuals perform everyday activities independently. They work with people of all ages, from children with developmental delays to older adults with age-related challenges.

Occupational therapy involves teaching adaptive techniques, recommending assistive devices, and modifying the environment to promote greater independence and quality of life.

3. Cognitive-Behavioral Therapy (CBT): CBT is a widely used form of psychotherapy that targets negative thought patterns and behaviors. It helps individuals identify and challenge irrational beliefs, manage stress, and develop healthier coping strategies. CBT is effective for various mental health conditions, including anxiety, depression, and PTSD.

4. Speech Therapy: Speech therapists, also known as speech-language pathologists, work with individuals who have speech, language, voice, or swallowing disorders. They employ exercises, communication

strategies, and assistive devices to improve communication skills and swallowing function.

5. Music Therapy: This therapy involves the use of music to address physical, emotional, cognitive, and social needs. Music therapists engage clients in activities such as listening to music, playing instruments, or songwriting to promote relaxation, emotional expression, and social interaction.

6. Art Therapy: Art therapists use various art forms to help individuals express themselves, explore emotions, and develop coping mechanisms. Through creating art, individuals can gain insights into their thoughts and feelings, leading to increased self-awareness and emotional healing.

7. ABA Therapy: Applied Behavior Analysis is an evidence-based intervention commonly used for children with autism spectrum disorder (ASD).

ABA therapy focuses on teaching skills, reducing challenging behaviors, and promoting positive behaviors through positive reinforcement and other behavior modification techniques.

8. Medication Management: For individuals with certain medical conditions, properly prescribed medications can be essential in managing symptoms, alleviating pain, and improving overall functioning. Regular follow-up with healthcare providers helps ensure proper dosage and effectiveness.

9. Support Groups: Support groups offer a safe and empathetic space for individuals facing similar challenges to share experiences, seek advice, and build a sense of community.

They can provide emotional support, reduce feelings of isolation, and help participants learn from one another's experiences.

10. Pain Management: Pain management techniques aim to reduce pain and improve daily functioning for individuals experiencing chronic or acute pain.

It can involve a combination of medications, physical therapy, relaxation techniques, and mindfulness practices to help individuals cope with and manage pain effectively.

11. Mindfulness and Meditation: Mindfulness practices involve being present in the moment without judgment, which can reduce stress and anxiety. Meditation techniques, such as deep breathing or guided imagery, can promote relaxation, improve focus, and enhance emotional well-being.

12. Animal-Assisted Therapy (AAT): AAT involves interactions with trained animals, such as dogs or horses, to promote emotional and physical healing.

 The presence of animals can reduce stress, anxiety, and loneliness, while encouraging social interactions and physical activity.

13. Social Skills Training: This intervention is beneficial for individuals with social difficulties, such as those with autism spectrum disorder or social anxiety.

Social skills training helps individuals improve communication, empathy, and relationship-building abilities, leading to increased social integration and self-confidence.

14. Nutritional Counseling: Proper nutrition plays a vital role in maintaining overall health and well-being.

Nutritional counseling can help individuals develop healthier eating habits, manage medical conditions, and achieve specific health goals.

15. Assistive Technology: Assistive technology includes devices, tools, and software designed to assist people with disabilities in performing tasks independently. Examples include hearing aids, screen readers for individuals with visual impairments, and adaptive keyboards.

16. Vocational Rehabilitation: Vocational rehabilitation programs support individuals with disabilities in developing skills and finding employment opportunities suited to their abilities. These programs aim to enhance employment prospects and foster greater financial independence.

17. Sensory Integration Therapy: This therapy benefits individuals with sensory processing disorders by helping them better process and respond to sensory information. Occupational therapists often use sensory integration techniques to improve sensory-related challenges.

18. Counseling and Psychotherapy: Beyond CBT, there are various other therapeutic approaches, such as psychodynamic therapy, person-centered therapy, and family therapy, each tailored to address different emotional and relational challenges.

19. Exercise and Physical Activity: Regular physical activity can have numerous benefits for overall health and well-being. It can improve mood, reduce stress, enhance cognitive function, and help manage various medical conditions.

20. Horticultural Therapy: This unique therapy involves engaging in gardening and plant-related activities to promote physical and emotional well-being. It can be particularly beneficial for individuals recovering from trauma, stress, or other mental health challenges.

Remember that the effectiveness of these therapies and interventions can vary depending on an individual's specific needs and circumstances. Therefore, it's essential to work with healthcare professionals to create a personalized plan that addresses the individual's unique challenges and goals, ultimately enhancing their quality of life.

It's important to note that the effectiveness of each therapy and intervention can vary depending on an individual's unique circumstances. A comprehensive approach, often involving multiple therapies and collaborative efforts among healthcare professionals, can lead to significant improvements in the individual's quality of life.

Chapter 8

Family Support and Advocacy: The Journey Together

Family Support and Advocacy: The Journey Together is a concept that emphasizes the importance of providing comprehensive support and advocacy for families facing various challenges. It aims to create a collaborative environment where families and professionals work together to address the unique needs of each family member and promote their well-being.

At its core, Family Support involves offering assistance, resources, and guidance to families dealing with issues such as parenting challenges, disabilities, mental health concerns, substance abuse, financial struggles, and other stressors that can impact family dynamics. This support can be provided through community-based programs, social services, counseling, and peer support groups.

Advocacy, on the other hand, involves actively championing the rights and interests of families within various systems and institutions. This may include advocating for better policies, access to services, and improved resources that can benefit families in need.

The journey together signifies the collaborative approach between families, service providers, and the wider community in working towards positive outcomes for families. It recognizes that each family's situation is unique, and therefore, personalized support and advocacy are essential.

Family Support and Advocacy: The Journey Together acknowledges that families are the primary support system for individuals, and nurturing healthy family dynamics is crucial for overall well-being. By promoting a strong network of support and advocating for systemic changes, it aims to strengthen families and contribute to healthier and more resilient communities.

Through this approach, families can find empowerment, guidance, and resources to navigate through challenging times and foster positive growth. Professionals, policymakers, and communities collectively play a vital role in this journey, ensuring that families receive the support and opportunities they need to thrive.

Family support and advocacy are two interconnected concepts that play essential roles in promoting the well-being of families, particularly those facing challenging situations or navigating complex systems. Here's a further explanation of each:

1.Family Support: Family support encompasses a broad range of interventions and services designed to assist families in various aspects of their lives. It recognizes that families are the foundation of society and that a nurturing and supportive family environment is crucial for the well-being and development of individuals, especially children.

a. Types of Family Support: Family support can take many forms, such as:

- Parenting Programs: Offering guidance and resources to parents to enhance their parenting skills and promote positive family dynamics.
- Financial Assistance: Providing aid to families facing economic challenges, ensuring their basic needs are met.
- Mental Health Services: Offering counseling or therapy for family members dealing with emotional or psychological issues.
- Healthcare Access: Facilitating access to medical services and resources for families to maintain their health.
- Educational Support: Providing educational resources and opportunities for children and adults alike.

b. Benefits of Family Support: Effective family support contributes to several positive outcomes:

- Improved Family Functioning: Families develop better communication, problem-solving, and coping skills, leading to healthier dynamics.

- Enhanced Child Development: Children benefit from stable and nurturing environments, leading to improved academic performance and social skills.

- Reduced Family Stress: Adequate support helps families handle life's challenges with more resilience and less stress.

- Strengthened Communities: Healthy families contribute to stronger, more cohesive communities.

2. Advocacy: Advocacy involves actively representing and promoting the rights, needs, and interests of families. It seeks to address systemic issues and barriers that hinder families from thriving and accessing necessary resources.

a. Types of Family Advocacy: Family advocates engage in various activities to effect change:

- Policy Advocacy: Lobbying for legislative changes and reforms to improve family-related laws and regulations.

- Awareness Campaigns: Raising public awareness about specific family issues, such as domestic violence or child welfare.

- Resource Mobilization: Advocating for increased
funding and support for family support programs
and services.

- Systemic Change: Working to address systemic
inequalities that disproportionately impact certain
families, like those from marginalized communities.

b. Importance of Family Advocacy: Effective family
advocacy is critical for several reasons:

- Amplifying Voices: Advocacy gives a voice to
families who may not have the means or platform to
express their concerns and needs.

- Creating Change: By addressing systemic issues,
advocacy can lead to broader, long-lasting
improvements in family well-being.

- Fostering Collaboration: Advocacy efforts often
involve collaboration with policymakers,
organizations, and communities to drive change.

The relationship between family support and advocacy is symbiotic. Family support services often benefit from advocacy efforts that secure funding and policy changes, enabling the provision of better support. Simultaneously, advocacy efforts are strengthened by demonstrating the importance and impact of family support services.

In conclusion, family support and advocacy are interconnected approaches aimed at creating supportive environments for families and empowering them to overcome challenges. By combining effective support services with targeted advocacy efforts, societies can better ensure the well-being and success of families, ultimately contributing to stronger and more cohesive communities.

Chapter 9

Education and Inclusion: Creating Supportive Environments

Education and inclusion involve creating supportive environments that ensure equal access and opportunities for all individuals, regardless of their diverse backgrounds, abilities, or identities. This approach aims to promote the participation, engagement, and success of every learner within the educational system. here are some comprehensive details on the topic:

Education and inclusion refers to the principles and practices that foster an inclusive learning environment, where all students, including those with disabilities, different cultural backgrounds, gender identities, and other unique traits, are welcomed, valued, and supported.

Importance of inclusive education is essential for several reasons.

- It promotes social cohesion.
- Reduces discrimination.
- Builds understanding and empathy among students.
- It also maximizes the potential of each individual, ensuring that no one is left behind in the learning process.

Key Elements of Creating Supportive Environments;

a. Accessible physical spaces: Ensuring that educational facilities are physically accessible to individuals with disabilities, including ramps, elevators, and appropriate classroom design.

b. Curriculum adaptation: Modifying teaching materials and methods to cater to diverse learning styles and abilities.

c. Inclusive pedagogy: Employing teaching strategies that encourage active participation and collaboration among students, accommodating different learning paces and preferences.

d. Support services: Providing additional support, such as learning aids, special educators, or interpreters, to assist students with specific needs.

e. Sensitivity and awareness: Promoting awareness and understanding of various cultures, disabilities, and identities within the school community to avoid biases and stereotypes.

f. Parent and community involvement: Engaging parents and the community to create a strong support system for inclusive education.

Benefits of Inclusion In Education;

a. Academic advantages: Inclusive environments have been shown to enhance academic performance for all students, as diverse perspectives and teaching approaches lead to a richer learning experience.

b. Social skills development: Interaction with peers from diverse backgrounds fosters social skills, empathy, and respect for differences.

c. Emotional well-being: Students feel more accepted and supported, leading to increased self-esteem and reduced feelings of isolation.

d. Preparation for real-world: An inclusive education prepares students to live and work in a diverse society, promoting tolerance and acceptance.

Challenges and Solutions;

a. Attitudinal barriers: Overcoming stereotypes and prejudices requires training and awareness campaigns for teachers, students, and the wider community.

b. Resource allocation: Inclusive education may require additional resources, but the long-term benefits justify the investment.

c. Teacher professional development: Providing teachers with adequate training in inclusive teaching methodologies is crucial for effective implementation.

Overall, Education and Inclusion: Creating Supportive Environments is a multifaceted approach that recognizes the uniqueness of each learner and aims to create an educational landscape where diversity is embraced, and all students can thrive and reach their full potential

1. Inclusive Education Strategies: Creating an inclusive educational environment involves implementing various strategies to accommodate diverse learners effectively. These strategies include:
   - Differentiated Instruction: Tailoring teaching methods and content to meet the individual needs, abilities, and learning styles of students.
   - Universal Design for Learning (UDL): Designing lessons and materials that are accessible and beneficial to all students, regardless of their abilities or backgrounds.
   - Collaborative Learning: Encouraging students to work together in diverse groups, fostering teamwork, and peer learning.

- Assistive Technology: Integrating technology tools and aids to support students with disabilities or specific learning needs.

- Individualized Education Plans (IEPs): Developing personalized educational plans for students with special needs, outlining specific goals and support services.

- Multicultural Education: Integrating diverse cultural perspectives and experiences into the curriculum to promote understanding and appreciation of different cultures.

2. Legal and Policy Framework: In many countries, inclusive education is supported by laws and policies that emphasize equal access to education. For instance, the United Nations Convention on the Rights of Persons with Disabilities (CRPD) calls for inclusive education, ensuring that individuals with disabilities have access to quality education on an equal basis with others. National laws and policies often provide guidelines for implementing inclusive practices in schools.

3. Collaboration and Involvement: Successful inclusive education requires collaboration among all stakeholders, including teachers, parents, students, administrators, and the community. By involving all parties, schools can identify the specific needs of students and create personalized support systems. Parent involvement is particularly critical, as they can provide valuable insights into their child's needs and advocate for their rights.

4. Teacher Professional Development: Teachers play a crucial role in creating inclusive environments. Providing them with ongoing professional development helps them build the skills, knowledge, and confidence necessary to support diverse learners effectively. This training may cover topics like understanding diverse learning needs, employing inclusive teaching methods, and promoting a positive and respectful classroom culture.

5. Continuum of Inclusion: Inclusion is not a one-size-fits-all approach. Instead, it follows a continuum, ranging from full inclusion, where all students are educated together in a mainstream classroom, to partial inclusion, where some students

receive certain services or support outside the regular classroom. The decision on the level of inclusion depends on the individual needs and abilities of each student.

6. Monitoring and Evaluation: Regular monitoring and evaluation of inclusive education practices are essential to assess their effectiveness and identify areas for improvement. Schools should collect data on student progress, engagement, and well-being to gauge the impact of inclusive initiatives and make data-driven decisions.

7. Barriers and Ongoing Challenges: Despite the benefits of inclusive education, there can be challenges in its implementation. Some common barriers include lack of funding, inadequate training, resistance to change, and societal attitudes towards disability and diversity. Addressing these challenges requires a commitment to continuous improvement and fostering a culture of inclusivity within educational institutions.

.

Chapter 10

Empowering Autistic Individuals: Embracing Diversity in Society

Embracing diversity in society is not only a moral imperative but also a gateway to building an inclusive and equitable world. Autistic individuals, just like any other person, have unique abilities, perspectives, and contributions that can enrich our communities if we create an environment that empowers and supports them. This comprehensive guide aims to shed light on the challenges faced by autistic individuals, highlight their strengths, and offer practical strategies to foster their empowerment and inclusion in society.

1. Understanding Autism:
- Defining autism spectrum disorder (ASD) and dispelling common myths.
- Highlighting the neurodiversity perspective and recognizing autism as a variation in human cognition.
- Discussing the diverse characteristics and challenges experienced by autistic individuals.

2. Challenging Stigma and Stereotypes:
- Addressing the harmful stereotypes and misconceptions surrounding autism.
- Promoting awareness and education to combat stigma and discrimination.
- Encouraging individuals to focus on abilities rather than limitations.

3. Empowering Autistic Individuals:
- Encouraging self-advocacy and empowering autistic individuals to speak up for their needs and rights.
- Providing support and resources to promote independence and autonomy.
- Promoting person-centered planning to ensure individualized support and accommodation.

4. Education and Employment:
- Advancing inclusive education practices that cater to the diverse learning needs of autistic students.
- Fostering a supportive and understanding work environment to enable autistic individuals to thrive professionally.
- Highlighting success stories of autistic individuals in various fields to inspire and promote equal opportunities.

5. Promoting Social Inclusion:
- Encouraging community engagement and creating opportunities for autistic individuals to socialize and build meaningful relationships.
- Training neurotypical peers and educators to be allies and understanding towards autistic individuals.
- Advocating for accessible public spaces and activities that cater to sensory sensitivities.

6. Mental Health and Well-being:
- Addressing mental health challenges faced by autistic individuals and promoting mental health awareness.

- Ensuring access to appropriate mental health services and support.
- Identifying coping strategies and self-care techniques for autistic individuals and their caregivers.

7. Family Support:
- Providing guidance and resources for families of autistic individuals to foster a nurturing and accepting home environment.
- Supporting parents and caregivers in understanding and responding to their child's unique needs.
- Connecting families with support groups and community networks to share experiences and knowledge.

8. Building Partnerships:
- Encouraging collaboration between the autism community, policymakers, educators, and businesses to create a more inclusive society.
- Promoting research and innovation to develop more effective support systems and interventions.
- Advocating for policy changes that protect the rights and welfare of autistic individuals.

Embracing diversity in society, especially when it comes to empowering autistic individuals, requires a collective effort from all members of the community. By challenging stereotypes, fostering inclusive education and workplaces, promoting social inclusion, and providing mental health support, we can create a world where autistic individuals can lead fulfilling lives, contribute to society, and be celebrated for their unique perspectives and talents. Together, we can build a society that values and embraces the diversity of all its members.

Conclusion

In conclusion, "Unraveling the Spectrum: Embracing the Brilliance of Autism" illuminates the beauty of diversity in human cognition. Through this journey, we have witnessed the incredible strengths and unique perspectives of individuals on the autism spectrum. Let us foster an inclusive society that values neurodiversity, empowering each person to shine their brightest. Together, we can create a world where everyone's brilliance is celebrated and embraced, making it a better and more harmonious place for all.

In closing, "Unraveling the Spectrum: Embracing the Brilliance of Autism" has been a captivating exploration into the multifaceted nature of autism. Throughout this journey, we have shattered misconceptions and biases, revealing the immense potential and gifts that individuals with autism bring to the world.

By recognizing and embracing the brilliance of autism, we can create a society that values every person for their unique abilities, irrespective of neurotypical norms. Let us cultivate an environment that fosters understanding, empathy, and support, enabling individuals on the spectrum to thrive and contribute meaningfully to our communities.

Together, we must champion inclusivity in education, employment, and social settings, ensuring that each person is given the opportunity to reach their fullest potential. Collaboration and acceptance will lead us to innovations and breakthroughs we could have never imagined.

As we move forward, let us remember that embracing the brilliance of autism is not just an act of kindness or charity; it is a celebration of the rich tapestry of humanity. It is an acknowledgment that our differences should be cherished and celebrated, for it is within this diversity that true progress and harmony lie.

In the spirit of empathy and compassion, let us stand united and committed to building a world where everyone's brilliance shines, no matter their place on the spectrum. Together, we can create a future where autism is not seen as a disability, but rather as a unique and essential aspect of our shared human experience.